Eosinophilic Esophagitis For Parents

Navigating EoE With This Comprehensive Handbook for Parents of Children with Eosinophilic Esophagitis.

Title:
Eosinophilic Esophagitis For Parents

Subtitle
Navigating EoE With This Comprehensive Handbook for Parents of Children with Eosinophilic Esophagitis.

Copyright © 2024 by (Dr. Joey Green)

Printed in the United States of America.

ISBN: 9798879683271

TABLE OF CONTENT

CHAPTER 1: INTRODUCTION TO EOSINOPHILIC ESOPHAGITIS

The condition known as eosinophilic esophagitis (EoE) is a persistent inflammatory condition that affects the esophagus. It is distinguished by the presence of an abnormally high number of eosinophils, which are a kind of white blood cell, in the tissue of the esophagus. EoE is a disorder that has only fairly recently been discovered, with the frequency and identification of the illness growing over the last few decades, particularly in youngsters. EoE has become a serious health problem owing to the impact it has on the quality of life of patients and the possible consequences that might arise if it is not addressed. This is even though it has only been recognized relatively recently.

What is Eosinophilic Esophagitis (EoE)?

Eosinophilic The main immunological response that causes esophagitis is inflammation and swelling of the esophageal lining, which is mediated by eosinophils. White blood cells called eosinophils are involved in allergy reactions as well as immunological responses against parasite infections. These eosinophils build up in the esophagus of people with eosinophil accumulation disorder (EoE), which causes inflammation, tissue damage, and further symptoms.

The chronic and recurring nature of EoE is one of its distinguishing characteristics. Over time, symptoms may wax and wane, and each person's experience with the disease's intensity may be different. EoE frequently manifests as dysphagia, chest discomfort, heartburn, regurgitation, nausea, and trouble swallowing meals. In addition to feeding issues, unwillingness to eat, and failure to flourish, children with EoE may also display behaviors that compromise their growth and development.

Causes and Risk Factors

Although the precise origin of the Epstein-Barr virus (EoE) is still unknown, it is thought to be complex, involving immunological dysregulation, environmental factors, and genetic predisposition. According to research, there may be a common immunological mechanism between EoE and allergy disorders such as atopic dermatitis, allergic rhinitis, and asthma.

Individuals are predisposed to EoE in part by genetic factors as well. A number of genes related to immune control and allergic reactions have been linked to the emergence of EoE. The intricate and incompletely understood relationship exists between environmental stimuli and genetic vulnerability.

For those who are vulnerable, environmental factors including exposure to certain allergens or food ingredients may cause or worsen symptoms of encephalitis (EoE). Food allergies including cow's milk, wheat, soy, eggs, and peanuts are frequently linked to EoE. Environmental allergens including pollen, dust mites, and animal dander, in addition to food allergies, may potentially play a role in the development of EoE or exacerbate symptoms in certain people.

Understanding the Impact on Children

Children's health and well-being can be significantly impacted by eosinophilic esophagitis, which can influence many areas of their everyday lives. A child's ability to eat can be severely hindered by the symptoms of Epstein-Barr syndrome (EoE), including difficulty swallowing, food aversion, and stomach pain. This can result in nutritional shortages, developmental delays, and other problems.

EoE children may have trouble eating, which can be upsetting for both the kid and their caretakers. These feeding issues might include gagging, choking, or vomiting during meals.

Due to their inability to eat with their classmates or participate in food-related social activities, children with feeding issues may experience mealtime conflicts, anxiety related to food, and social isolation.

Furthermore, the necessity for continuous medical care and the chronic nature of EoE can cause disruptions in children's and families' everyday lives. The emotional and practical burden of the condition may be increased by frequent doctor's appointments, food restrictions, and medical procedures that interfere with family routines, extracurricular activities, and school attendance.

Moreover, it is important to recognize the psychological effects of having a chronic condition like EoE. Due to their symptoms and dietary limitations, children with EoE may feel frustrated, embarrassed, or low in self-esteem. They could also experience anxiety or sadness as a result of their medical condition and how it affects their day-to-day activities.

CHAPTER 2: SIGNS AND SYMPTOMS OF EOE

A kind of white blood cell called an eosinophil counts abnormally high in the esophageal tissue, which is indicative of a chronic inflammatory condition of the esophagus known as eosinophilic esophagitis (EoE). The signs and symptoms of Epstein-Barr syndrome might fluctuate greatly between people and age groups. Understanding the telltale signs and symptoms of endometriosis (EoE) is essential for prompt diagnosis and suitable treatment. We will look at common symptoms in kids, their causes, and how symptoms might change with maturity in this extensive overview.

Common Symptoms in Children

Eosinophilic Children with esophagitis may exhibit a wide range of symptoms, varying in intensity and length. When a kid has EoE, common symptoms include:

1. Difficulty Swallowing (Dysphagia): Children with EoE may have trouble swallowing, commonly known as dysphagia. They may feel as if food is trapped in their throat or chest, causing discomfort or anguish while swallowing. Dysphagia can cause extended meal times, reluctance to eat, and avoidance of specific food textures.

2. Food impaction happens when a piece of food becomes trapped in the esophagus, resulting in an obstruction. Children with EoE may have recurring episodes of food impaction, which can be unpleasant and upsetting. Food impaction may necessitate immediate medical intervention to clear the blockage and relieve symptoms.

3. Heartburn and Chest Discomfort: Children with EoE may suffer from gastroesophageal reflux disease (GERD), which causes heartburn and chest pain. These symptoms may be aggravated by the inflammation and constriction of the esophagus caused by EOE. Children may report a burning feeling

in the chest or upper abdomen that intensifies after eating or lying down.

4. Regurgitation is the involuntary movement of stomach contents, including food and drink, back into the esophagus or mouth. Children with EoE may have regurgitation due to reduced esophageal motility or reflux symptoms. Regurgitation can occur spontaneously or be prompted by specific meals or activities.

5. Children with EoE may feel nausea or vomiting, especially after eating. Dysphagia, food impaction, and reflux symptoms can all cause nausea and vomiting. These symptoms can significantly affect a child's

appetite, nutritional intake, and general quality of life.

6. Feeding Difficulties: Children with EoE may have feeding issues, such as refusing to eat, gagging, or choking during meals. Dysphagia, fear of food impaction, or an intolerance to specific textures or tastes can all cause feeding difficulties. If not addressed, children may avoid particular meals or food categories, which can lead to nutritional deficits and development delays.

7. Failure to Thrive: In severe cases of EoE, children may have failure to thrive, which is defined as insufficient weight gain or

development below the normal trajectory for their age and gender. Failure to thrive can be caused by feeding issues, nutritional malabsorption, or higher energy expenditure as a result of the inflammatory response associated with EoE. Early detection and management are critical to avoiding long-term consequences caused by failure to thrive.

8. Other Symptoms: In addition to the frequent symptoms listed above, children with EoE may have stomach discomfort, bloating, diarrhea, or constipation. These symptoms might be vague and overlap with other

gastrointestinal illnesses, making diagnosis difficult.

It is significant to remember that children's presentations of EoE can differ greatly, and not everyone will have the same collection of symptoms. While some kids may only occasionally or mildly have symptoms, others may have severe or ongoing symptoms that call for medical attention. Furthermore, without careful assessment and observation, symptoms may change over time, making it difficult to get a firm diagnosis.

Recognizing Potential Triggers

Managing the illness and minimizing symptom exacerbations require identifying probable causes for EoE symptoms. Common EoE triggers include the following, however individual triggers may differ.

1. Food Allergens: For many people, food allergies are a key cause of EoE symptoms. Cow's milk, wheat, soy, eggs, peanuts, tree nuts, fish, and shellfish are common dietary allergies linked to EoE. To determine which particular food allergens are causing their symptoms, children with EoE may be subjected to allergy testing, such as blood or skin prick tests.

2. Environmental Allergens: In addition to food allergies, certain people may have worsening symptoms of allergic eczema due to environmental allergens such as mold, dust mites, pollen, and animal dander. These allergens have the potential to cause an allergic reaction in the esophagus, which can result in inflammation and flare-ups of symptoms.

3. Dietary Factors: For some people, eating spicy or acidic meals, and drinking carbonated drinks, coffee, or alcohol might exacerbate their symptoms of eating disorders. These food triggers have the potential to worsen inflammation and irritate the lining of the esophagus,

increasing the risk of dysphagia, heartburn, or chest discomfort.

4. Physical Irritants: Apart from dietary variables and allergens, physical irritants can cause symptoms of early onset eosinophilia (EoE), including food impaction and dysphagia. These include extremes in temperature, big food particles, and sharp objects. It may be beneficial for kids with EoE to change their eating habits or diet to reduce their exposure to physical allergens.

5. Stress and Worry: For certain people, emotional stress and anxiety can worsen the symptoms of Epstein-Barr syndrome.

Hormones linked to stress can affect the immune system and gastrointestinal motility, which may exacerbate inflammation and symptom severity. Stress-reduction strategies for kids with EoE might include support groups, therapy, and relaxation exercises.

Identifying and avoiding possible triggers for symptoms of Epstein-Barr syndrome is crucial for treating the illness and enhancing the quality of life for those who are impacted. Maintaining a thorough symptom journal and collaborating closely with medical professionals can assist in pinpointing certain triggers and creating individualized treatment plans.

How Symptoms Vary Across Age Groups

Age-related variations in anatomy, physiology, and dietary habits can be reflected in the presentation of eosinophilic esophagitis. It's critical to comprehend how symptoms may differ between age groups to accurately diagnose and treat EoE. Here, we go over how EoE often manifests in newborns, kids, teens, and adults:

1. Infants and Toddlers: Nonspecific symptoms include feeding issues, irritability, failure to thrive, and frequent vomiting can be seen in infants and toddlers with early onset of EoE. During bottle or nursing, infants may show signs of difficulty swallowing, gagging, or

choking. They could also get intolerant to particular flavors or textures in food or develop a food aversion. One typical consequence of epilepsy in babies is failure to grow, which is caused by insufficient intake and absorption of nutrients.

2. Children: As children become older, their EoE symptoms—such as dysphagia, food impaction, heartburn, chest discomfort, regurgitation, and stomach pain—may become more noticeable and prominent. When swallowing, children may experience feeling as though food gets caught in their chest or throat, causing pain or discomfort. If treatment is not received, feeding issues

and food aversion may worsen and lead to malnutrition and delayed growth.

3. Teens: Teens with Epstein-Barr syndrome (EoE) may encounter symptoms such as dysphagia, heartburn, chest discomfort, regurgitation, and abdominal pain that are common in children and adults. Teenagers may, however, also display extra signs of puberty and hormonal changes, such as irregular menstruation, mood swings, or exhaustion. Adolescents with EoE may also have varying degrees of symptom intensity and coping strategies due to psychological reasons including stress or body image issues.

4. Adults: Dysphagia, food impaction, heartburn, chest discomfort, regurgitation, and stomach pain are among the symptoms of eoe that adults may experience. Adults may, however, also exhibit unusual or coexisting symptoms of GERD, such as persistent coughing, hoarseness, or clearing of the throat. Adults with EoE may also have symptoms for a longer period and be more likely to develop problems like Barrett's esophagus or esophageal strictures.

CHAPTER 3: DIAGNOSIS AND TESTING

A complete strategy is required to diagnose eosinophilic esophagitis (EoE). This method consists of a full clinical evaluation, diagnostic tests, and a histological analysis of esophageal tissue. As a result of the general character of EoE symptoms and the fact that they overlap with symptoms of other gastrointestinal illnesses, it can be difficult to arrive at a conclusive diagnosis. Within the scope of this all-encompassing guide, we will investigate the path to diagnosis, the function of endoscopy and biopsy procedures, as well as other diagnostic tests that are utilized in the assessment of endo-esophageal esophagitis (EoE).

Steps to Diagnosis

Examining the Eosinophilic System These are the standard stages involved in the treatment of esophagitis:

1. Clinical Assessment: A comprehensive clinical evaluation, comprising a full medical history and physical examination, is the first step in the diagnostic procedure. Medical professionals will question the patient's symptoms, including their length, intensity, and possible causes. In addition, they will check for allergies, underlying medical issues, and a family history of EoE or other allergy disorders. To evaluate EoE, a thorough dietary history that includes any

food allergies or intolerances is also necessary.

2. Symptom Assessment: Medical professionals will evaluate the patient's symptoms, which may include dysphagia (difficulty swallowing), regurgitation, heartburn, chest discomfort, nausea, vomiting, stomach pain, or trouble feeding. To direct additional diagnostic tests and treatment, it is critical to distinguish the symptoms of EoE from those of GERD or other gastrointestinal illnesses.

3. Elimination diets: To find possible food triggers for EoE symptoms, medical professionals may occasionally advise an

elimination diet. Elimination diets include cutting out particular food categories or allergens from the diet for a while, then gradually reintroducing them to see whether the symptoms return. Dietary management techniques can be guided by elimination diets, which can assist in identifying food allergies causing EoE.

4. Allergy testing: To pinpoint certain food allergens or environmental allergens that are causing symptoms of environmental allergies, allergy testing may be carried out. Patch testing, serum IgE testing, and skin prick testing are examples of allergy testing methodologies. For individuals with EoE,

recognizing and avoiding allergens can help lessen symptom exacerbations and enhance results.

5. Testing for Eosinophilic Esophagitis: Endoscopic assessment and histological analysis of esophageal tissue are commonly used in diagnostic testing. Direct esophageal viewing and biopsy sample collection for histological examination are made possible by endoscopy. Additional diagnostic procedures, including imaging investigations or testing for esophageal motility, could be carried out to look for problems or related illnesses.

Endoscopy and Biopsy Procedures

An essential diagnostic tool for assessing Eosinophilic Esophagitis is endoscopy, which enables direct sight of the esophagus mucosa and the biopsy sample collection for histological examination. The techniques for endoscopy and biopsy used to diagnose EoE are as follows:

1. Preparation: To guarantee the stomach is empty, patients are advised to fast for a predetermined amount of time before the surgery. To guarantee the patient's comfort throughout the surgery, sedation or anesthesia may be given. All drugs, especially blood thinners and anticoagulants, which may need to be temporarily stopped,

should be disclosed to the patient's healthcare practitioner.

2. Endoscopic Evaluation: An endoscope, which is a flexible tube equipped with a light and camera, is introduced through the mouth and gradually advanced down the esophagus during an endoscopic operation. With the use of an endoscope, a medical professional can view the esophagus mucosa and look for indications of edema, inflammation, constriction, or other anomalies. To find any abnormalities, the whole length of the esophagus is extensively inspected.

3. Biopsy Sampling: Using specialized forceps, many biopsy samples are taken from the esophagus mucosa during endoscopy. To guarantee representative sampling, biopsy samples are taken from the esophagus's normal- and abnormal-appearing regions. The distal (lower) and proximal (upper) esophagus are the usual places from which biopsy samples are taken to look for variations in eosinophilic inflammation across regions.

4. Histological Examination: A pathologist processes biopsy samples and looks at them under a microscope to check for eosinophils and other histological characteristics that are specific to EoE. Eosinophilic When there are

more than 15 eosinophils per high-power field in the esophageal epithelium, it is considered esophagitis. To confirm the diagnosis of EoE, the histological investigation also looks for other inflammatory alterations such as subepithelial fibrosis, dilated intercellular gaps, and basal cell hyperplasia.

5. Histological Confirmation: The presence of eosinophilic inflammation in the esophageal mucosa is necessary for the diagnosis of eosinophilic esophagitis. The diagnosis of esophageal eosinophilia (EoE) is supported by a biopsy sample that shows an elevated number of eosinophils in the absence of

other potential explanations (such as reflux esophagitis or infection).

The most reliable method for determining the severity of Eosinophilic Esophagitis and making a diagnosis is still endoscopy combined with biopsy. To differentiate eosinophilic inflammation (EoE) from other causes of esophageal eosinophilia and to inform suitable therapy methods, histological confirmation of eosinophilic inflammation is crucial.

Other Diagnostic Tests and Their Importance

Other diagnostic tests may be carried out in addition to endoscopy and biopsy procedures to assess individuals with Eosinophilic Esophagitis for complications or related disorders. These examinations might consist of:

1. Imaging Investigations: To check for structural irregularities, strictures, or motility issues in the esophagus, imaging studies like barium swallow or esophagram may be carried out. Swallowing a contrast substance that covers the esophagus and makes its structure and function visible on X-ray pictures is known as a barium swallow.

2. Testing for Esophageal Motility: This test can be used to look for abnormalities in the function of the esophagus, such as dysmotility disorders or esophageal dysmotility. To gather data on the motility and function of the esophagus, esophageal manometry analyzes the pressure and coordination of esophageal muscle contractions.

3. pH Monitoring: In individuals exhibiting symptoms of erosion of the stomach, pH monitoring may be carried out to screen for acid reflux or gastroesophageal reflux disease (GERD). Ambulatory pH monitoring uses a pH probe that is put into the

esophagus to assess the frequency and length of acid reflux episodes throughout 24 hours.

4. Blood Tests: In individuals with Eosinophilic Esophagitis, blood tests may be carried out to check for indicators of inflammation, allergies, or nutritional deficiencies. Complete blood counts (CBCs), serum IgE levels, allergy panels, and testing for certain nutritional deficiencies are examples of blood tests that may be performed (e.g., iron deficiency anemia).

5. Skin Testing: In individuals with EoE, skin prick or patch testing may be used to determine if they have become sensitized to

certain food allergens or environmental allergens. To find possible triggers for EoE symptoms, skin testing is putting tiny quantities of allergen extracts into the skin and monitoring the skin's response.

These diagnostic tests may offer further details on the severity, complications, or comorbidities of the disease, and they serve a supplementary role in the assessment of eosinophilic esophagitis. Accurate diagnosis and treatment of EoE need a thorough diagnostic strategy that includes clinical assessment, endoscopy with biopsy, and ancillary tests.

CHAPTER 4: TREATMENT OPTIONS

A chronic inflammatory condition of the esophagus called eosinophilic esophagitis (EoE) is defined by an abnormally high concentration of eosinophils in the esophageal tissue. The goals of managing esophageal reflux disease (EoE) are to lessen symptoms, decrease esophageal inflammation, avoid complications, and enhance the lives of those who are impacted. Medication, new treatments, and dietary control are available for treating early-onset EoE. We will examine the several approaches to treating EoE in this extensive guide, including pharmacological interventions, dietary modifications, and novel therapeutics.

Dietary Management: Elimination of Diets and Food Allergies

Since many people with eosinophilic esophagitis (EoE) have underlying food allergies or sensitivities that exacerbate their symptoms, dietary management is essential to the treatment of EoE. The treatment of EoE may involve the adoption of the following nutritional strategies:

1. Elimination Diets: To discover and get rid of probable triggers for symptoms of Epstein-Barr syndrome, elimination diets entail cutting out particular food categories or allergies from the diet. Cow's milk, wheat, soy, eggs, peanuts, tree nuts, fish, and shellfish are common allergies linked to EoE.

Under the supervision of a licensed dietitian or healthcare professional, elimination diets can be used to guarantee sufficient nutrition and avoid nutritional shortages. Elimination diets have varying degrees of success in easing symptoms of eating disorders, and they may need to be carefully monitored and adjusted over time.

2. Elemental Diet: This type of eating obviates exposure to allergens in food by supplying all necessary nutrients in a predigested form through the use of a hypoallergenic formula. Elemental formulas are appropriate for people with numerous food allergies or severe EoE since they are usually devoid of common food allergens and are amino acid-

based. Elemental diets can be employed as a short- or long-term therapeutic approach to reduce inflammation in the esophagus and EoE symptoms.

3. The six main dietary allergens—milk, cow's wheat, soy, eggs, peanuts, and seafood—are to be eliminated from the diet according to the empirical Six-Food Elimination Diet (SFED). Removing the most prevalent dietary triggers for EOE is the foundation of SFED, which has been proved to be beneficial in causing remission of EOE symptoms in certain people. To assist long-term dietary control and identify particular food allergens

contributing to EoE, SFED may be utilized as a diagnostic technique.

4. Diets aimed at eliminating certain food allergens found by allergy testing or food trials are called allergen-specific elimination diets, and their effect on symptoms of inflammatory bowel disease (EoE) is evaluated by cutting these allergens out of the diet. To identify and remove trigger foods, allergen-specific elimination diets can be led by skin prick tests, serum IgE testing, patch testing, or oral food challenges. These diets are customized for each person based on their unique food sensitivities and may

call for close observation and dietary adjustments.

5. Targeted Food Exclusion: In order to lessen EoE symptoms, targeted food elimination is removing particular trigger items from the diet that have been found by symptom tracking or food experiments. Meals that trigger reactions might vary from person to person and can include typical food allergies, foods that are acidic or hot, or foods with certain textures or consistencies. To reduce symptom exacerbations and enhance quality of life, targeted food exclusion seeks to identify and steer clear of particular dietary triggers.

To create individualized dietary programs, track symptom response, and guarantee appropriate nutrition, dietary treatment of end-of-life illness (EoE) necessitates close collaboration between patients, healthcare practitioners, and registered dietitians. To improve outcomes for people with EoE, long-term dietary management techniques may include dietary adjustments, periodic food reintroduction challenges, and continuous monitoring of symptoms and nutritional status.

Medications and Their Role

Medication is an important aspect of the therapy of Eosinophilic Esophagitis, especially for those whose symptoms are resistant or chronic. Dietary control is also important. The following drugs can be used to treat EoE:

- Proton Pump Inhibitors (PPIs): PPIs are frequently used to treat GERD or gastroesophageal reflux disease, and they may also be useful in easing the symptoms of EoE in certain people. PPIs reduce the production of stomach acid, which helps lessen the symptoms of reflux, chest discomfort, and heartburn that are related to EoE. For EoE, PPIs are usually used as first-line treatment in conjunction with dietary control.

- Topical Steroids: The cornerstone of pharmacologic therapy for Eosinophilic Esophagitis is topical steroids, such as ingested corticosteroid formulations. Topical drugs enhance symptoms and histologic results by decreasing eosinophilic infiltration and esophageal inflammation. Metered-dose inhalers or nebulizers are used to provide ingested corticosteroids, such as fluticasone or budesonide, directly to the esophageal mucosa, where they are swallowed without being absorbed into the bloodstream. For those with EoE who don't improve with diet and PPI medication, topical steroids are usually used as a second-line treatment.

- Systemic Steroids: In situations of severe or resistant eosinophilic esophagitis, systemic steroids, such as prednisone or prednisolone, may be used as a short-term therapy. Systemic steroids have the potential to cause weight gain, mood swings, osteoporosis, and immunological suppression, but they are also useful in lowering esophageal inflammation and bringing about a clinical remission of EoE symptoms. Systemic steroids are not advised for long-term maintenance therapy; instead, they are usually used for short-term induction therapy or in cases of acute exacerbations of EoE.

- Biotherapies: As a promising therapy option for patients with severe or refractory illness, biologic treatments that target certain immune pathways implicated in Eosinophilic Esophagitis are beginning to emerge. Biomarkers that limit eosinophilic inflammation and lower esophageal eosinophil levels, including anti-interleukin-5 (IL-5) monoclonal antibodies (like mepolizumab, reslizumab) or anti-interleukin-4/13 monoclonal antibodies (like dupilumab), ameliorate symptoms and histologic results. Clinical studies are also being conducted to assess biologic medicines, which might provide an alternate course of treatment for EoE patients who do not react to traditional treatments.

- **Other Drugs:** In the treatment of eosinophilic esophagitis, other drugs such as mast cell stabilizers, leukotriene receptor antagonists, or immunomodulators may be utilized, especially in patients with coexisting allergies or refractory symptoms. These drugs can be used as supplementary therapy in conjunction with topical steroids and dietary control since they target different immunological pathways implicated in the pathophysiology of EoE.

Drugs are essential for the treatment of Eosinophilic Esophagitis because they reduce inflammation in the esophagus, relieve symptoms, and guard against consequences. The intensity of the symptoms, the patient's reaction to the first course of treatment, and other considerations all play a role in the prescription decision. Maintaining close observation and scheduling routine check-ups with medical professionals are necessary to maximize drug therapy and reduce adverse effects.

Innovative Therapies and Emerging Treatments

Novel therapy and developing treatments are being studied for the management of Eosinophilic Esophagitis, in addition to dietary control and medication. These treatments give patients with refractory or severe illness alternate choices by focusing on particular immunological pathways implicated in the pathophysiology of EoE. Here are a few instances of cutting-edge therapies and new treatments for EoE:

1. Biologic Medicines: As a possible treatment for patients with severe or refractory illness, biologic therapies that target certain immunological pathways linked to

eosinophilic esophagitis are being researched. Anti-interleukin-5 (IL-5) and anti-interleukin-4/13 monoclonal antibodies are examples of biologic medicines that suppress eosinophilic inflammation and lower esophageal eosinophil levels, improving histologic findings and symptoms. Clinical studies are presently being conducted to assess biologic treatments, which might provide a different course of treatment for patients who do not respond to traditional medications.

2. Anti-Siglec-8 Antibodies: The cell surface receptor Siglec-8, which is expressed on mast cells and eosinophils, is involved in controlling eosinophilic inflammation.

Researchers are looking at anti-siglec-8 antibodies as possible therapeutic agents to treat eosinophilic esophagitis. By blocking the activation of eosinophils and mast cells' Siglec-8 receptors, these antibodies lessen esophageal inflammation. Preclinical and clinical trials are presently being conducted to assess anti-Siglec-8 antibodies for the treatment of EoE.

3. Topical Immunotherapy: To promote tolerance and desensitization to certain dietary allergens, topical immunotherapy entails administering allergen-specific immunotherapy directly to the esophagus mucosa. The goals of topical immunotherapy are to lessen eosinophilic inflammation and

regulate the immune response in the esophagus. Different topical immunotherapy modalities, including epicutaneous immunotherapy (EPIT) and sublingual immunotherapy (SLIT), are being studied as possible treatments for eosinophilic esophagitis.

4. Microbiome Modulation: Immune system regulation and mucosal homeostasis maintenance are significantly influenced by the gut microbiome. Eosinophilic esophagitis etiology has been linked to dysbiosis or changes in the makeup of the gut microbiome. Probiotics, prebiotics, and fecal microbiota transplantation (FMT) are a few examples of microbiome modification

techniques that are being researched as possible EoE treatment methods. The goals of these therapies are to support immunological tolerance to food antigens and restore the balance of microbes in the gut.

5. Gene therapy: To modify gene expression and improve therapeutic results, genetic material is delivered to specific cells or tissues. Gene therapy, which targets certain genes implicated in immune dysregulation or allergic reactions, shows promise as a viable therapeutic option for Eosinophilic Esophagitis. To lessen eosinophilic inflammation and enhance clinical results,

immune cell modifications or alterations to gene expression in the esophagus are being investigated using gene editing techniques like CRISPR-Cas9.

Novel therapeutic approaches for developing treatments for Eosinophilic Esophagitis have the potential to enhance treatment results and broaden the range of alternatives available to patients with severe or refractory symptoms. Intending to provide individualized, precision medicine methods for the therapy of EoE, these medications target certain immunological pathways implicated in the etiology of EoE. To assess these innovative medicines' long-term effects, safety, and effectiveness in people with

EoE, more investigation and clinical studies are

required.

CHAPTER 5: LIFESTYLE ADJUSTMENTS AND COPING STRATEGIES

Eosinophilic esophagitis (EoE) is a chronic inflammatory esophageal disorder that can have a major effect on an afflicted person's everyday life as well as their emotional health and that of their family. In addition to medical care, managing end-of-life issues involves modifying one's lifestyle and developing coping mechanisms to get over obstacles and preserve one's standard of living. This thorough guide will go over coping mechanisms for the emotional toll that EoE has on everyday life, as well as options for parents and families to seek out assistance.

Practical Tips for Managing Daily Life

Inhabiting an Eosinophilic To reduce symptoms and maximize well-being, esophagitis demands making realistic modifications to daily routines, food habits, and social activities. Here are some useful hints for adjusting to everyday life with EoE:

1. Dietary Modifications: To identify and eliminate trigger foods that worsen EoE symptoms, adhere to a strict elimination diet or dietary restrictions as advised by medical professionals or trained dietitians. To monitor symptoms and pinpoint possible trigger foods, keep a food journal. When dining out, let caregivers, family members, and restaurant employees know about any

dietary restrictions. Also, plan your meals and snacks ahead of time.

2. Meal Preparation: To satisfy dietary requirements and guarantee food safety, adjust cooking and food preparation processes. Steer clear of items that are tough to swallow or might lead to food impaction and choose instead for gentler textures. Try different recipes and ingredients to make tasty, allergy-free meals that yet satisfy your needs.

3. Portion Manage: To reduce pain and lessen symptoms of reflux or dysphagia, control your portion sizes and refrain from overindulging. Instead of eating big, hefty

meals throughout the day, eat smaller, more frequent ones. To aid in swallowing and digesting, chew meals well and take tiny pieces.

4. Hydration: Make sure you are getting enough water throughout the day. Drink non-acidic liquids to reduce esophageal discomfort, such as water, herbal teas, or diluted fruit juices. Steer clear of alcohol, coffee, and carbonated beverages since these might make reflux symptoms worse.

5. Mealtime Ambience: Establish a tranquil, stress-free atmosphere during mealtimes that won't interfere with eating. Make time

for meals and snacks, and concentrate on indulging in food and interacting with family members. Reduce the amount of time you spend distracted by electronics, TV, or work-related activities when eating.

6. Chewing and Swallowing Techniques: To avoid choking or food impaction, practice chewing food completely and swallowing it gently. Chew food gently and in tiny, manageable portions to facilitate digestion and lower the risk of dysphagia. Steer clear of chatting or laughing while eating, since this might make it more likely that food would lodge in the esophagus.

7. Safe Eating Procedures: To avoid contamination and foodborne disease, pay attention to food safety and hygiene procedures. Before handling food, make sure your hands are completely clean. You should also make sure your surfaces, cutting boards, and kitchen equipment are cleaned. Perishable goods should be carefully stored to preserve freshness and safety. Adhere to suggested storage rules.

8. Travel and Eating Out: Make advance plans for travel and eating out to guarantee that safe, allergy-free food alternatives are available. Consult restaurant menus ahead of time and let the staff know about any dietary needs or food allergies. For ease of

eating on the go, bring along portable meals or snacks. In addition, pack any essential prescriptions or emergency supplies in case of unintentional exposure.

Strategies for Coping with Emotional Impact

Individuals and their families may have severe emotional effects, such as stress, worry, frustration, and social isolation, as a result of living with eosinophilic esophagitis. Resilience, support, and self-care techniques are necessary for overcoming the emotional difficulties of an End-of-Earth crisis and preserving mental and emotional health. The following are methods for managing the emotional toll that EoE has on one's life:

1. Knowledge and Awareness: Gain knowledge about Eosinophilic Esophagitis and its causes, symptoms, available treatments,

and prognosis for yourself and your family members. Seek trustworthy information from respected sources, including peer-reviewed publications, patient advocacy groups, and healthcare practitioners. Being aware of the nature of the illness might make people feel less afraid and more empowered to take an active role in their treatment.

2. Encourage candid and open dialogue about your experiences, worries, and needs about end-of-life with loved ones, caregivers, and medical professionals. Openly communicate your thoughts and feelings, and invite others to do the same and provide their support. In managing EoE, effective communication may

promote cooperation, trust, and relationship building.

3. Seek emotional assistance from friends, family, support organizations, or mental health specialists who are aware of the difficulties associated with having eosinophilic esophagitis. Join social media groups or online forums for people with EoE and their families to meet others, talk about experiences, and discuss coping mechanisms. Join support groups or therapy sessions to get advice, affirmation, and inspiration from people going through comparable struggles.

4. Self-Care Routines: Make self-care routines a priority to maintain your emotional, mental, and physical health and lower your stress levels. Take part in joyful, calming, and fulfilling pursuits, such as yoga, meditation, physical activity, hobbies, or artistic endeavors. To develop awareness, acceptance, and resilience in dealing with the unknowns and difficulties of living with end-of-life experiences, practice mindfulness practices.

5. Develop constructive coping mechanisms to handle the stress, worry, and unpleasant feelings brought on by eosinophilic esophagitis. Utilize adaptive coping

strategies, cognitive reframing, and problem-solving techniques to transform negative feelings and ideas into productive and upbeat viewpoints. Keep your attention on the things you can manage, and be proactive in addressing problems and coming up with solutions.

6. Seek Professional Help: Seek professional assistance from a qualified mental health professional, such as a psychologist, psychiatrist, or counselor, if you are finding it difficult to manage the emotional effects of EoE or if you are exhibiting symptoms of anxiety, depression, or other mental health issues. In a secure and encouraging setting,

therapy or counseling may help you examine your emotions, build coping mechanisms, and discover practical methods for handling stress and emotional discomfort.

7. Family Support: To guarantee a cooperative and encouraging approach, involve family members, particularly parents and caregivers, in the care and management of eosinophilic esophagitis. Family members should be encouraged to communicate openly, to actively participate, and to support one another. They should also work as a team to tackle the duties and obstacles that come with managing EoE. Acknowledge and value the assistance that your family has

provided for your mental and physical health.

8. Establish Reasonable Expectations: When it comes to the management of eosinophilic esophagitis and how it affects day-to-day living, establish reasonable expectations for both yourself and your loved ones. Realize that there may be ups and downs, obstacles, and setbacks when dealing with a chronic health condition like EoE. On the path to improved health and wellbeing, remember to be kind, patient, and forgiving to both yourself and other people. You should also rejoice in your little successes.

Support Resources for Parents and Families

Access to peer support networks, educational resources, and support services can help parents and families of children with eosinophilic esophagitis manage the difficulties of raising a child with a chronic illness. Support options for parents and families impacted by EoE include the following:

1. Patient Advocacy Groups: Establish contact with organizations that support patients with eosinophilic esophagitis, such as the Campaign Urging Research for Eosinophilic Disease or the American Partnership for Eosinophilic Disorders (APFED) (CURED). For

people and families impacted by EoE, these organizations offer priceless resources, instructional materials, support services, and advocacy campaigns.

2. Online Support Groups: To connect with other families, share experiences, exchange information, and get advice from peers going through similar struggles, parents of children with eosinophilic esophagitis should join online support groups or forums. Parents may ask for concerns, look for advice, and get emotional support from people who understand the effects of EoE on family life in safe and empathetic online groups.

3. Parent Education Programs: To learn more about Eosinophilic Esophagitis (EoE), its management, and methods for assisting children with EoE, take part in parent education programs, workshops, or webinars provided by healthcare practitioners, patient advocacy groups, or community organizations. Parent education programs equip parents with essential information, abilities, and tools to support their child's health and wellbeing.

4. Family Counseling: To address the emotional and relational dynamics within the family system and improve family support, communication, and cohesiveness, think

about family counseling or therapy. Family counseling can improve resilience in handling stress and uncertainty, assist parents and siblings cope with the difficulties of living with eosinophilic esophagitis, and help them create coping mechanisms.

5. Educational Assistance: To make sure that accommodations and support are in place to meet academic and social needs connected to Eosinophilic Esophagitis, work closely with your child's school, teachers, and educational support agencies. To provide a secure and welcoming learning environment for your child, inform school staff about your

kid's health, dietary requirements, and any necessary adjustments or changes.

6. Engage in peer mentorship programs or make connections with other families who have dealt with children diagnosed with eosinophilic esophagitis. Based on their personal experiences overcoming the difficulties of EoE, peer mentors can offer insightful advice, useful hints, and emotional support. Programs for peer mentorship enable families impacted by EoE to assist and share information.

7. Community Resources: Learn about the recreational opportunities, support services,

and community resources that are accessible to families with children who have specific healthcare requirements, such as eosinophilic esophagitis. Families impacted by long-term medical illnesses may be able to take advantage of activities, events, and services provided by nearby community centers, religious institutions, and community-based support groups.

8. Respite Care: Make arrangements for parents and other caregivers to receive short-term relief so they may relax, refuel, and take care of their self-care requirements. To give parents and other caregivers a break and avoid burnout,

respite care services offer qualified caregivers who can help with child care, monitoring, and support for kids with special healthcare needs.

CHAPTER 6: NAVIGATING THE HEALTHCARE SYSTEM

Building a supportive medical team, communicating effectively with healthcare personnel, and standing up for your child's needs are all important aspects of navigating the healthcare system when dealing with Eosinophilic Esophagitis (EoE). The long-term management and care coordination of esophageal inflammation, or EoE, are necessary. We will discuss how to navigate the healthcare system with EoE in this extensive guide. Some of the tactics we will cover include creating a supportive medical team, communicating effectively with healthcare personnel, and speaking up for your child's needs.

Building a Supportive Medical Team

For your kid to get thorough treatment and effectively manage Eosinophilic Esophagitis, you must assemble a supportive medical team. The complicated requirements of people with EoE can be met by a multidisciplinary approach including different healthcare practitioners, specialists, and allied health workers. The following important individuals make up the medical team that treats children with EoE:

- A pediatric gastroenterologist is a physician who focuses on the identification and management of gastrointestinal issues in children. As specialists in diagnosis, therapy planning, and long-term care methods, pediatric gastroenterologists are essential to the management of eosinophilic esophagitis.

- A physician who specializes in the diagnosis and treatment of immunological disorders and allergic illnesses is known as an allergist/immunologist. In particular, they are invaluable in recognizing and treating food allergies or sensitivities that may exacerbate the symptoms of early onset encephalitis (EoE).

- A registered dietitian is a medical practitioner who specializes in dietetic management and nutrition. To ensure that people with eating disorders get enough of the necessary nutrients while avoiding trigger foods, registered dietitians collaborate closely with people who have eating disorders and their families to create individualized dietary plans, offer nutrition counseling, and track nutritional status.

- Pediatrician/Family Physician: In addition to organizing general healthcare and preventative services, a pediatrician or family physician acts as the child's main care physician when it comes to Eosinophilic Esophagitis. Pediatricians are essential in treating comorbid diseases, keeping an eye on development, and offering families impacted by EoE continuous assistance and direction.

- Speech-Language Pathologist: Speech-language pathologists are experts in diagnosing and treating speech-language deficits as well as swallowing difficulties (dysphagia). For children with EoE, speech-language pathologists evaluate swallowing function, give swallowing treatment, and suggest ways to enhance oral intake and mealtime safety.

- Psychotherapist/Counselor: For people and families dealing with long-term medical disorders like Eosinophilic Esophagitis, a psychologist or counselor offers psychological treatments, counseling, and emotional support. Psychologists assist kids and families in managing the psychological effects of early exposure to events, addressing stresses, and creating coping mechanisms to improve resilience and overall wellbeing.

- Care Coordinator/Case Manager: The role of a care coordinator or case manager is to act as an intermediary between families, community resources, and healthcare practitioners to streamline care delivery, organize services, and attend to both practical and psychological needs. Care coordinators assist and advocate for families impacted by EoE, help families navigate the healthcare system, and schedule appointments.

- Developing cooperative relationships with medical professionals, encouraging candid communication, and actively taking part in shared decision-making about your child's care are all important components of building a supportive medical team. When medical professionals collaborate, they can offer children with eosinophilic esophagitis comprehensive, patient-centered treatment that is customized to meet their specific requirements.

Effective Communication with Healthcare Providers

Promoting excellent outcomes and maximizing treatment for children with eosinophilic esophagitis need effective communication between the patient and the healthcare professional. Families and healthcare providers may make shared decisions by fostering mutual understanding, trust, and open and honest communication. The subsequent tactics are recommended for proficient communication with healthcare providers:

1. Organize Your Questions and Concerns: Make a list of the questions, issues, and symptoms you would like to discuss with your healthcare professional before your visit. To share with healthcare professionals,

bring pertinent medical documents, test results, and prescription lists. Make a documented inventory of all the drugs, vitamins, and dietary supplements your child is taking at the moment, together with the doses and schedule for administration.

2. Ask Questions: Get information from medical professionals about your child's diagnosis, available treatments, and prognosis. During appointments, take notes or ask a friend or family member to go with you and assist you capture information. Never be afraid to ask for clear answers in plain language, as well as for other resources or recommendations if you need more knowledge.

3. Communicate Your Worries: Be open and truthful with healthcare professionals about your concerns, preferences, and care objectives for your kid. Inform us of any changes in your child's health or well-being-related symptoms, habits, or overall quality of life. Take the initiative to speak up for your child's needs and preferences, and work with medical professionals to create a customized care plan.

4. Seek Second Views: If you're having trouble managing your eosinophilic esophagitis, think about consulting or getting second opinions from other medical professionals, experts, or university medical facilities. When treating your child's illness, second

views can offer insightful analysis, different viewpoints, and other treatment alternatives to take into account.

5. Use Telehealth Services: To speak with healthcare practitioners remotely, especially for routine follow-up appointments, medication management, or symptom monitoring, make use of telehealth services, virtual consultations, or telemedicine platforms. Telehealth services provide fast, convenient, and accessible healthcare without requiring in-person visits.

6. Follow-Up and Follow-Through: Consult your doctor again if necessary for routine checkups, prescription modifications, or

additional testing. Follow treatment advice, dietary guidelines, and lifestyle adjustments given by medical professionals. To guarantee continuity of treatment and the best possible therapy for eosinophilic esophagitis, keep note of visits, prescription refills, and suggested follow-up care.

For children with eosinophilic esophagitis, optimal outcomes need joint decision-making, trust-building, and effective communication with healthcare professionals. Families may guarantee thorough, patient-centered care catered to their child's specific needs by actively engaging in conversations, raising questions, voicing concerns, and working together with healthcare providers.

Advocating for Your Child's Needs

To guarantee that children with eosinophilic esophagitis have access to the right treatment, resources, and support services, you must speak out for their needs. You are your child's best advocate and voice in the medical system as a parent or caregiver. Here are some tactics to help you speak out for your child's needs:

- Learn About Eosinophilic Esophagitis: Get knowledgeable about the causes, signs, and treatments of this condition as well as management techniques. Seek trustworthy information from respected sources, including peer-reviewed publications, patient advocacy groups, and healthcare practitioners. Being aware of your child's condition helps you make wise decisions and successfully represent them in court.

- Effective Communication: Maintain open lines of communication with educators, healthcare professionals, and other parties engaged in your child's care. Clearly state the symptoms, treatment preferences, medical history, and care objectives for your kid. Make sure that your child's voice is heard and valued during decision-making processes by politely but firmly advocating for their needs and rights.

- Work Together with Healthcare Professionals: Work together with healthcare professionals to create a customized care plan that is suited to your child's unique requirements, preferences, and objectives. Engage in active participation in care conversations, pose inquiries, and offer feedback on treatment choices. To maximize your child's health and wellbeing, fight for their access to the right medical care, therapies, and support resources.

- Seek Accommodations: To address your child's educational, social, and developmental requirements connected to Eosinophilic Esophagitis, advocate for accommodations and support services. Create a 504 plan, also known as an individualized education plan (IEP), in close collaboration with your child's educators, educational support services, and school. This plan should include accommodations and adjustments that will support your child's academic performance and overall well-being.

- Access Support Services: Families impacted by eosinophilic esophagitis should look for access to community resources, support groups, and support services. To network with other families, exchange stories, and gain access to peer support and informative resources, get in touch with patient advocacy groups, internet forums, or neighborhood support groups.

- Raise Awareness: To help lawmakers, the public, and healthcare professionals better understand and recognize eosinophilic esophagitis, advocate for more funding for research, education, and awareness campaigns. Talk about your child's experience, spread the word on social media, and take part in advocacy campaigns to push for better care and support services for people with end-of-life issues.

- Participate in Advocacy Activities: Engage in grassroots campaigns and advocacy efforts to push for legislation, funding for research, and policy changes that will enhance the treatment and assistance provided to people with eosinophilic esophagitis. To lobby for policy reforms that address the needs of persons with EoE, one can interact with elected officials, participate in advocacy campaigns, and join patient advocacy organizations.

It takes perseverance, tenacity, and cooperation with educators, healthcare professionals, and community stakeholders to advocate for your child's needs. You can make sure your kid gets the resources, care, and support they need to flourish despite the difficulties associated with having eosinophilic esophagitis by actively advocating on their behalf.

CHAPTER 7: EDUCATION AND SCHOOL SUPPORT

To manage their health condition and achieve academic achievement, children with Eosinophilic Esophagitis (EoE) depend heavily on education. Children with EoE and their families may have particular difficulties navigating the school system, but with good teamwork, modifications, and assistance, kids may succeed both academically and socially. This extensive book will cover methods for collaborating with educators and schools, securing accommodations via 504/IEP plans, and assisting kids with emotional and behavioral difficulties to thrive in social and academic contexts.

Working with Schools and Educators

Supporting children with Eosinophilic Esophagitis in the educational context requires cooperation between families, medical professionals, and school staff. Parents and teachers can collaborate to establish a nurturing atmosphere that caters to the special requirements of kids with EoE. The following are some methods for collaborating with educators and schools:

1. Open Contact: Make sure you have open lines of communication with all the staff members at your child's school, including the teachers, counselors, and nurses. Tell the teachers about your child's diagnosis of early

onset epilepsy (EoE), symptoms, treatment plan, dietary restrictions, and any adjustments or changes that may be required.

2. Inform School Personnel: Provide education to school staff regarding Eosinophilic Esophagitis, including its causes, signs, and triggers in addition to management techniques. Give school staff educational resources, such as fact sheets, pamphlets, or presentations, to assist them in comprehending how EoE affects your child's health and academic achievement.

3. Create a Health Plan: Create a comprehensive health plan, also known as an individualized healthcare plan (IHP), in collaboration with the school nurse or health services team. This plan should detail your child's medical needs, emergency procedures, medication administration techniques, and dietary restrictions. Make sure that everyone who needs to know at the school is aware of the health plan and knows what to do in an emergency.

4. Coordinate Care: To guarantee continuity of treatment and support for your child's medical needs throughout school hours, coordinate care between healthcare

professionals and school staff. To promote cooperation and well-informed decision-making, communicate with school personnel as required on your child's medical history, treatment updates, and any changes in their health.

5. Defend adolescents with chronic health issues like eosinophilic esophagitis by advocating for a safe, inclusive school atmosphere that fosters acceptance, empathy, and respect. This will help combat bullying and stigma. To create anti-bullying rules and educational programs that will increase awareness and promote an inclusive culture, collaborate with school

administration to address bullying, taunting, or prejudice linked to your child's condition.

6. Take Part in School Activities: To foster socialization, peer connection, and involvement in the school community, encourage your kid to take part in clubs, events, and school activities. To guarantee your child's complete participation in and access to extracurricular activities, fight for any necessary adjustments or changes.

7. Attend Meetings: To discuss your child's accomplishments, academic objectives, and support needs, attend school meetings such as parent-teacher conferences, Section 504

plan meetings, and Individualized Education Program (IEP) meetings. Speak out in favor of adjustments, changes, or extra services to meet your child's specific learning requirements and guarantee academic achievement.

Accommodations and 504/IEP Plans

To meet their health-related requirements and promote their academic progress, children with eosinophilic esophagitis may need accommodations or adaptations in the educational environment. Section 504 plans, accommodations, and Individualized Education Programs (IEPs) can offer a framework for guaranteeing that kids with EoE get the tools and support they need to succeed in school. The following are typical accommodations and methods for securing 504/IEP plans:

1. **504 Plan:** For children with disabilities or long-term health issues that significantly impair one or more key living activities,

including eating or learning, a Section 504 plan is a legally binding document outlining accommodations, modifications, and support services. To provide equitable access to school and meet the special requirements of children with EoE, a 504 plan offers a blueprint.

Examples of 504 Plan Accommodations for EoE:

- Allow for regular potty breaks or access to restroom facilities as needed.

- Permission to bring water or oral hydration products to remain hydrated during the school day.

- If symptoms interfere with attention or productivity, allow for extra time to complete assignments, tests, or classwork.

- Changes in classroom seating arrangements to meet dietary requirements or reduce exposure to probable allergies.

- Establish a dedicated safe place or quiet area for pupils to relax or manage symptoms during the school day.

2. **Individualized Education Program (IEP):** An Individualized Education Program (IEP) is a tailored education plan created for children with disabilities or special needs who need specialized instruction, support

services, or accommodations to access the curriculum and advance in school. Children with Eosinophilic Esophagitis may be eligible for an IEP if their condition adversely affects their academic performance or educational development.

Components of an IEP for EoE:

- Academic goals are tailored to the student's specific requirements, abilities, and areas for progress.
- Specialized teaching, accommodations, and support services are provided to help students meet their learning requirements and achieve academic achievement.

- Speech therapy, occupational therapy, and counseling are examples of related treatments that may be provided to address the educational impact of EoE on the development and functioning of students.

- Transition planning and goal setting help students prepare for postsecondary education, vocational training, employment, or independent life.

3. **504/IEP Meetings:** Attend 504 plan or IEP meetings with school professionals, including teachers, administrators, special education staff, and other service providers, to review your child's needs, objectives, and support

services. Advocate for adjustments, modifications, and services that meet your child's health requirements while still promoting academic achievement. Review and update the 504 plan or IEP regularly to ensure that it accurately represents your child's changing needs and progress.

4. **Documentation and Medical Records:** Document your child's Eosinophilic Esophagitis diagnosis, medical history, treatment plan, and functional restrictions to help build a 504 plan or IEP. Collaborate with healthcare providers, therapists, and other experts to gather relevant medical records, assessments, and evaluations that document

your child's requirements and help offer appropriate accommodations and services.

Helping Your Child Thrive Academically and Socially

To help students with Eosinophilic Esophagitis in the social and academic facets of school life, parents, teachers, and support agencies must work together proactively. Children with EoE can flourish in the classroom and reach their full potential if their social and intellectual needs are met. The following are some tips to support your child's social and intellectual development:

Establish Reasonable Expectations: Considering your child's aptitudes, interests, and preferred method of learning, establish reasonable expectations for their academic performance. Prioritize effort, growth, and advancement over merely achieving academic goals. Both within and outside of the classroom, encourage your kid to follow their hobbies, discover new interests, and feel proud of their accomplishments.

Promote Academic Support: To meet your child's learning requirements and encourage academic achievement, promote academic support services like tutoring, remedial teaching, or enrichment activities. Collaborate with educators, special education personnel, and support services to create customized approaches and interventions that focus on your child's unique problem areas.

Encourage Self-Advocacy: Give your kids the tools they need to successfully communicate their needs, preferences, and accommodations to classmates, teachers, and other school staff. Urge your kid to speak out, to ask for assistance when necessary, and to firmly advocate for any adjustments or accommodations that may enhance their learning and overall well-being.

Promote Peer Interaction: Motivate your kids to socialize with others, take part in group activities, and form good relationships with their classmates both within and outside of the school. Give your kids the chance to interact with their peers, join organizations or extracurricular activities, and form friendships based on similar experiences and interests.

Encourage Your Kid to Take Ownership of Their Learning, Arrange Their Schoolwork, Manage Their Time Well, and Advocate for Their Needs on Their Own: These actions will help your child develop independence and self-management skills. Encourage your kid to make decisions, solve issues, and face obstacles head-on by giving them the support and direction they need when required.

Encourage Positive Coping Strategies: Instruct your kid in the use of positive coping mechanisms to deal with stress, worry, or discomfort brought on by scholastic pressures or eosinophilic esophagitis. Encourage your kid to use mindfulness exercises, relaxation methods, or creative outlets to help them manage stress, become more resilient, and maintain emotional health.

Celebrate Your Child's Academic Success: Acknowledge and honor your child's academic accomplishments, no matter how minor. Acknowledge their efforts, advancement, and tenacity in overcoming barriers or difficulties associated with eosinophilic esophagitis. Honor their tenacity, willpower, and fortitude in the face of difficulty and in accomplishing their objectives.

CHAPTER 8: LONG-TERM OUTLOOK AND PROGNOSIS

The buildup of eosinophils, a kind of white blood cell, in the esophageal tissue is the hallmark of Eosinophilic Esophagitis (EoE), a chronic inflammatory illness of the esophagus. Even though EoE is regarded as a chronic disorder, several variables might affect its long-term outlook and prognosis, such as the intensity of symptoms, how well the therapy works, and whether or not there are any coexisting conditions. We will discuss the chronic nature of EoE, the value of monitoring and follow-up treatment, current research advancements, and potential future avenues in EoE management in this extensive guide.

Understanding the Chronic Nature of EoE

Eosinophilic Esophagitis is a chronic illness that usually lasts a long time and needs constant care to manage symptoms, avoid complications, and achieve the best possible long-term results. In contrast to acute diseases that might go away on their own or with short-term care, EoE often has a chronic course marked by recurring bouts of inflammation and symptom flare-ups. The underlying immunological dysregulation and genetic susceptibility that cause persistent inflammation and tissue damage in the esophagus are the causes of the chronic character of esophageal reflux disease (EoE).

Key aspects of understanding the chronic nature of EoE include:

- Recurrence of Symptoms: People with encephalitis (EoE) are more likely to experience recurring bouts of symptoms such as dysphagia, which is trouble swallowing food, chest discomfort, heartburn, and reflux. With time, these symptoms may wax and wane, with remission intervals interspersed by flare-ups brought on by dietary changes, environmental allergies, or other causes.

- Illness Progression: Over time, EoE may result in fibrosis, scarring, and constriction of the esophagus, particularly in cases of chronic, untreated, or poorly managed disease. Food impaction, difficulty swallowing, and problems like esophageal rips (perforation) or structuring-related crises can all be caused by esophageal strictures.

- Effect on Quality of Life: Due to the chronic nature of EoE, afflicted persons and their families may experience physical discomfort, dietary restrictions, social limits, and mental suffering, all of which can have a substantial negative influence on their quality of life. To deal with the difficulties and uncertainties that come with having a chronic health condition like EoE, one must practice constant management, adaptability, and resilience.

- Multifactorial Management: Treating end-of-life symptoms while addressing the underlying inflammation requires a multifactorial strategy. Individualized lifestyle alterations, pharmaceutical therapy, endoscopic procedures, and dietary modifications are some examples of treatment techniques.

Even though EoE is regarded as a chronic disorder, proactive treatment techniques can assist afflicted people in maintaining better long-term results by reducing inflammation, controlling symptoms, and controlling their symptoms. To effectively manage end-of-life outcomes and maximize long-term prognosis, routine monitoring and follow-up treatment are crucial.

Monitoring and Follow-Up Care

To manage Eosinophilic Esophagitis over the long term, monitoring and follow-up care are essential because they allow medical professionals to evaluate the disease's activity, track the effectiveness of treatment, and make necessary adjustments to management plans. Frequent follow-up consultations provide the continuous assessment of symptoms, endoscopic observations, and esophageal tissue histological alterations. Important components of tracking and post-exposure management in EoE comprise:

- Clinical Evaluation: Perform routine clinical assessments to evaluate general health, growth metrics in children, nutritional status, and symptoms. Ask about any changes in your quality of life, eating habits, medication compliance, and symptoms since your last appointment. Conduct a thorough physical examination, making sure to evaluate the abdomen, neck, and oropharynx.

- Endoscopic Evaluation: To gauge the degree of esophageal inflammation, track mucosal alterations, and assess the efficacy of treatment, do routine endoscopic assessments, such as esophagogastroduodenoscopy (EGD) with esophageal biopsy. Gather many esophageal biopsy samples from both the proximal and distal locations to provide representative tissue samples for histological examination.

- Histological Assessment: Determine additional histopathological characteristics suggestive of EoE and evaluate esophageal biopsy specimens histologically to quantify eosinophilic inflammation, and examine for signs of tissue remodeling (e.g., fibrosis, basal zone hyperplasia). Track alterations in epithelial architecture, inflammatory infiltrates, and eosinophil counts over time to assess the state of the illness and the effectiveness of therapy.

- Objective Measures: To evaluate esophageal function, assess for comorbid conditions (e.g., gastroesophageal reflux disease), and identify potential triggers or contributing factors to EoE symptoms, consider adjunctive diagnostic modalities such as esophageal impedance-pH monitoring, esophageal manometry, or allergy testing.

- Treatment Modification: Depending on the patient's reaction to therapy, the level of disease activity, and the desired course of treatment, management techniques can be modified with the use of monitoring and follow-up evaluations. Treatment plans should be customized to target symptom alleviation, mucosal healing, and preventing long-term consequences related to EoE.

- Promote interdisciplinary cooperation amongst gastroenterologists, allergists, dietitians, speech-language pathologists, and other medical professionals who treat individuals with Epstein-Barr syndrome. To give impacted people comprehensive, coordinated management, coordinate care, exchange information, and incorporate treatment suggestions.

Optimal long-term results for persons affected by Eosinophilic Esophagitis need regular monitoring and follow-up therapy. Healthcare practitioners can customize management methods to meet the changing requirements of patients with end-of-life experience and to support the best possible health and well-being by closely monitoring disease activity, treatment reactions, and potential consequences.

Research Advances and Future Directions

Research breakthroughs have deepened our knowledge of Eosinophilic Esophagitis and opened the door for novel treatment and diagnostic strategies meant to enhance the prognosis of those who are afflicted. The pathophysiology of EoE is still being investigated, new biomarkers are being found, and tailored treatments are being developed to address the underlying immunological dysregulation and inflammation connected to the disorder. Important developments in EoE research and future directions include:

- Genetic Studies: Look into the genes that are susceptible to Eosinophilic Esophagitis, its genetic variations, and the molecular pathways that are involved in the etiology of the illness. Next-generation sequencing methods and genome-wide association studies (GWAS) are employed to clarify the genetic makeup of EoE and pinpoint possible treatment targets.

- Investigate the immune processes that underlie eosinophilic esophagitis. T-helper cell subsets, cytokines, chemokines, and inflammatory mediators are some of the factors that contribute to eosinophilic inflammation and esophageal tissue destruction. Clinical studies are being conducted to study targeted immunomodulatory medicines to modify immunological responses and restore immune tolerance.

- The goal of biomarker discovery is to find and confirm indicators of disease activity, response to therapy, and progression of eosinophilic esophagitis. Biomarkers are substances that may be used in clinical practice to help with diagnosis, monitoring, and prognostication. Examples of biomarkers include blood-based markers, tissue-based markers, imaging biomarkers, and non-invasive assessments of disease activity.

- Personalized medicine: Create Eosinophilic Esophagitis treatment plans that are unique to each patient and take into account their traits, disease phenotypes, biomarker profiles, and response to therapy. Precision medicine tactics are designed to reduce treatment-related side effects, enhance therapeutic results, and customize treatment regimens to each patient's unique requirements and preferences.

- Biologic Therapy: Assess the safety and effectiveness of biologic therapies that target certain immunological pathways, such as interleukin (IL)-5, IL-13, or immunoglobulin E, that are thought to be involved in the pathophysiology of eosinophilic esophagitis (IgE). Targeted reduction of eosinophilic inflammation and adjustment of immunological responses in EoE is possible using biological medicines.

- Investigate new drug delivery methods, formulations, or apparatuses to deliver therapeutic agents to the esophagus in a focused manner. This will increase the effectiveness of the medication, lower systemic exposure, and minimize off-target effects. Oral formulations, topical sprays, or esophageal stents that are intended to provide drugs directly to the afflicted mucosa are examples of localized drug delivery techniques.

- Research on Patient-Centered Outcomes: Examine how Eosinophilic Esophagitis affects quality of life, functional status, psychological well-being, and use of healthcare resources. To make sure that research goals and outcomes are in line with the needs and preferences of patients with end-of-life experience, consider patient-reported outcomes, caregiver views, and stakeholder involvement in clinical research projects.

Discoveries in the field of eosinophilic esophagitis might revolutionize our knowledge of the illness and enhance the lives of those who suffer from it. Researchers seek to improve the long-term prognosis and quality of life for patients with this chronic inflammatory condition by addressing unmet needs in EoE care, applying customized therapeutic methods, and bringing scientific findings into clinical practice.

CHAPTER 9: STORIES OF HOPE AND RESILIENCE

For people and families, living with Eosinophilic Esophagitis (EoE) can mean a variety of obstacles, from navigating the healthcare system and coping with the emotional effects of the illness to managing symptoms and dietary limitations. Notwithstanding these difficulties, a great number of EoE-affected people and families exhibit incredible fortitude, bravery, and tenacity in the face of hardship. We will examine first-hand narratives from families dealing with early-life experiences in this extensive book, as well as motivational tales of overcoming obstacles, finding hope, and fostering resilience within the EoE community.

Personal Accounts from Families Living with EoE

Families dealing with eosinophilic esophagitis frequently experience ups and downs, successes and disappointments, happiness, and hardships. Every family's experience with end-of-life effects is distinct and influenced by personal circumstances, viewpoints, and coping mechanisms. Through sharing their own stories, families impacted by EoE may help, uplift, and stand with other families going through comparable struggles. Here are a few first-hand stories from families experiencing EoE:

- **The Smith Family:**

When Ethan, the Smith family's youngest kid, began having frequent episodes of trouble swallowing, stomach pain, and food impaction, the family's adventure with EoE officially began. At the age of five, Ethan received a diagnosis of Eosinophilic Esophagitis following many medical visits and diagnostic testing. The family was first taken aback by the diagnosis, but they soon came together to study EoE, look into treatment possibilities, and modify their way of life to meet Ethan's nutritional needs.

Notwithstanding the difficulties in coping with EoE, the Smith family has drawn resilience and strength from their common experiences. They now act as ambassadors for EoE awareness, taking part in fundraising campaigns, support groups, and community activities to spread the word and encourage more research. The Smith family's journey has taught them the value of open communication, cooperation, and unwavering love in conquering the difficulties associated with having eosinophilic esophagitis.

- **The Patel Family:**

The Patel family's experience with EoE started when their three-year-old daughter, Maya, was given an Eosinophilic Esophagitis diagnosis. Maya's symptoms, which included trouble swallowing, an unwillingness to eat, and frequent vomiting fits, raised questions about her general health and nutritional state. The

Patel family's journey changed when their daughter was diagnosed with EoE. They sought out specialist treatment, made connections with other families impacted by the condition, and spoke out for their daughter's needs.

The Patel family has persevered and found hope in their daughter's tenacity and will, despite the early difficulties in handling EoE. With bravery and elegance, Maya has accepted her dietary limitations and discovered inventive ways to indulge in her favorite meals while avoiding trigger foods that worsen her symptoms. Despite the difficulties of having eosinophilic esophagitis, Maya can function well because of the assistance of her family, medical professionals, and neighborhood services.

- **The Johnson Family:**

The Johnson family's experience with eating disorders started when their seven-year-old son, Jacob, began exhibiting symptoms of reflux, chest discomfort, and trouble swallowing. Following many consultations with pediatricians, gastroenterologists, and allergists, an endoscopic biopsy revealed that Jacob had Eosinophilic Esophagitis. The Johnson family originally found the diagnosis to be daunting, but they moved swiftly to become knowledgeable about EoE, look into possible treatments, and speak out for their son's needs.

The Johnson family has persevered in handling the effects of EoE while maintaining optimism and resilience by leaning on their shared experiences, faith, and support system. Making connections with other families impacted by EoE, exchanging resources, and sharing encouraging and hopeful anecdotes has given them comfort. The Johnson family has gained important insight into fortitude, tenacity, and the strength of the community in overcoming the difficulties associated with living with eosinophilic esophagitis throughout their experience.

These first-hand narratives shed insight into the range of feelings, experiences, and difficulties that families dealing with eosinophilic esophagitis deal with. These families show bravery, resiliency, and steadfast drive in the face of adversity, despite the challenges they have faced. Through sharing their experiences, they provide others going through a similar journey with EoE motivation, encouragement, and support.

Inspiring Stories of Overcoming Challenges

Apart from first-hand narratives from families affected by Eosinophilic Esophagitis, there are several motivational tales of people who, despite having EoE, have surmounted obstacles, defied expectations, and accomplished amazing feats. For anyone going through similar challenges, these stories may be a source of inspiration, hope, and motivation. The following are some motivational tales of people who overcame obstacles related to eosinophilic esophagitis:

- **Sarah's Story:**

At 10 years old, Sarah began to have severe abdomen pain, trouble swallowing, and food impaction. Her doctor diagnosed her with Eosinophilic Esophagitis. Even though treating EoE might be difficult, Sarah didn't allow it to stop her from going after her goals in life or from being who she was. Sarah followed her passion for music and performance, becoming a skilled singer-songwriter and EoE awareness champion with the help of her family, medical team, and local resources.

Sarah has encouraged people impacted by chronic illnesses to never give up hope by sharing her own story with others, advocating for Eosinophilic Esophagitis, and spreading awareness of the disease via her music. Sarah is strong, tenacious, and appreciative of the chances she has to change the world despite the obstacles she encounters.

- **Michael's Story:**

As a teenager, Michael had dysphagia, food impaction, and esophageal strictures. He was diagnosed with Eosinophilic Esophagitis. Michael refused to allow EoE to control his destiny or break his spirit, even despite the physical restrictions placed on him by his disease. Michael followed his love of athletics and became a successful athlete and motivational speaker with the help of his family, friends, and medical professionals.

Through his accomplishments in sports and public speaking, Michael has motivated others with long-term medical illnesses to keep going, get over setbacks, and face life's difficulties head-on with bravery and fortitude. Michael continues to be upbeat, resolute, and appreciative of the chances he has to inspire people and change the world despite the obstacles he has encountered.

- **Emily's Story:**

Emily faced difficulties with dysphagia, dietary limitations, and social isolation after receiving a diagnosis of Eosinophilic Esophagitis as a young adult. Emily refused to allow her disability to define her or restrict her potential despite the challenges she faced. Through the encouragement of her loved ones, medical staff, and online community, Emily followed her dream of becoming a published writer and EoE awareness champion.

Emily has shared her personal story with others, encouraged people going through similar struggles, and increased awareness of the effects of Eosinophilic Esophagitis on individuals and families through her writing and advocacy efforts. Emily is resilient, imaginative, and driven to positively impact the lives of those impacted by EoE despite the uncertainty she encounters.

These motivational tales of people who have surmounted obstacles related to eosinophilic esophagitis serve as a reminder of the strength of fortitude, tenacity, and optimism in the face of difficulty. These people have persevered, followed their passions, and improved the world despite the challenges they have faced. They provide those going through similar difficulties with EoE hope, support, and inspiration via their tales.

CONCLUSION

In conclusion, living with eosinophilic esophagitis (EoE) presents a multitude of challenges for individuals and families. These challenges include the management of symptoms and dietary restrictions, as well as the navigation of the healthcare system and the management of the emotional impact of the condition. Many individuals and families that are impacted by EoE exhibit incredible resilience, tenacity, and endurance in the face of hardship. This is even though they are confronted with severe obstacles. Shared experiences provide the EoE community with a source of hope, solidarity, and strength. This is accomplished via the sharing of personal anecdotes and motivational tales of overcoming obstacles. By sharing their experiences, people and families who are impacted by eosinophilic esophagitis (EoE) can provide support, encouragement, and inspiration to others who are going through similar things. This serves to remind them that they are not alone in their journey with eosinophilic esophagitis.

APPENDIX

Dietary changes are frequently necessary to identify and avoid trigger foods that worsen symptoms and esophageal inflammation in the management of eosinophilic esophagitis (EoE). EoE-friendly recipes and wholesome, well-balanced meal plans may help families and individuals manage the difficulties of having an eating disorder while also allowing them to enjoy delectable, fulfilling meals. We offer sample meal plans and dishes in this appendix that are specific to people who have eosinophilic esophagitis.

<h1 style="text-align:center">Sample Meal Plan:</h1>

Note: Only for illustration reasons, this sample meal plan should be modified to account for personal dietary preferences, dietary sensitivity, and food allergies.

Breakfast:

- Almond milk oatmeal topped with sliced bananas and honey drizzle.
- Eggs cooked in a scramble with feta cheese, tomatoes, and spinach.
- Herbal tea or infused water.

Morning Snack:

- Almond butter and cut strawberries paired with rice cakes.

- Hummus on sticks with carrots.

- Tea is made with herbs or water.

Lunch:

- Mixed greens, cherry tomatoes, cucumber, avocado, and balsamic vinaigrette topped with grilled chicken salad.

- Rice pilaf or quinoa paired with sautéed veggies (bell peppers, zucchini, onions).

- Sparkling water or water with mint and lemon infusions.

Afternoon Snack:

- Granola and honey paired with Greek yogurt.

- Almond butter atop apple slices.

- Herbal tea or infused water.

Dinner:

- Fish baked in a lemon-dill sauce.
- Cauliflower and broccoli cooked under steam.
- Sweet potatoes roasted.
- Herbal tea or sparkling water.

Evening Snack:

- Rice pudding flavored with raisins and cinnamon.
- Nutritional yeast seasoned popcorn.
- Tea made with herbs or water.

EoE-Friendly Recipes:

1. Baked Chicken Parmesan:

Ingredients:

- Boneless, skinless chicken breasts

- Gluten-free breadcrumbs

- Olive oil

- Salt, pepper, Italian seasoning

- Grated Parmesan cheese

- Marinara sauce (look for brands without added spices or allergens)

Instructions:

- Turn the oven on to 375°F, or 190°C.

- Combine breadcrumbs, grated Parmesan cheese, Italian seasoning, salt, and pepper in a shallow dish.

- Dredge the chicken breasts in the breadcrumb mixture and press firmly to bind.

- Arrange the chicken breasts on a parchment paper-lined baking pan.

- Drizzle chicken breasts with olive oil.

- Bake the chicken for 25 to 30 minutes, or until it's golden brown and cooked through.

- Accompany with roasted veggies or gluten-free spaghetti and marinara sauce.

2. Quinoa Salad with Lemon-Herb Vinaigrette:

Ingredients:

Red onion, thinly sliced

Kalamata olives, pitted

Cooked quinoa

Mixed greens (spinach, arugula, kale)

Cherry tomatoes, halved

Cucumber, diced

Feta cheese, crumbled (optional)

For the Lemon-Herb Vinaigrette:

- Dijon mustard

- Garlic, minced

- Fresh herbs (parsley, basil, dill), chopped

- Salt and pepper to taste

- Fresh lemon juice

- Extra-virgin olive oil

Instructions:

- Cooked quinoa, mixed greens, cherry tomatoes, cucumber, red onion, and Kalamata olives should all be combined in a big dish.

- To create the vinaigrette, combine the lemon juice, olive oil, Dijon mustard, minced garlic, fresh herbs, salt, and pepper in a small container.

- After adding the vinaigrette, mix the quinoa salad to ensure uniform coating.

- If desired, sprinkle crumbled feta cheese on top.

- Serve cold as a wholesome and revitalizing salad substitute.

Appendix B: Frequently Asked Questions (FAQs)

For those who have Eosinophilic Esophagitis (EoE), as well as their families, living with the illness frequently brings up a lot of questions and worries. Answering commonly asked questions (FAQs) can help people navigate the difficulties of EoE by offering clarification, direction, and support. We answer frequently asked issues concerning the treatment of eosinophilic esophagitis in this appendix.

1. What is Eosinophilic Esophagitis (EoE)?

Eosinophilic A kind of white blood cell called an eosinophil buildup in the esophageal tissue is a characteristic of esophagitis, a chronic inflammatory illness of the esophagus. Chest discomfort, heartburn, food impaction, and trouble swallowing are some of the symptoms associated with EOE.

2. Which factors typically cause eosinophilic esophagitis?

Food allergies (dairy, wheat, soy, eggs, nuts), environmental allergens (pollen), acid reflux, and several drugs are common causes of allergic eoedema (EoE). One key to controlling Epstein-Barr syndrome is recognizing and avoiding trigger foods.

3. How does one diagnose eosinophilic esophagitis?

Eosinophilic A combination of clinical assessment, endoscopic examination (esophagogastroduodenoscopy, or EGD), and histological study of esophageal biopsy specimens is usually used to diagnose esophagitis. Eosinophilic inflammation, mucosal rings or furrows, and tissue remodeling are examples of characteristic findings.

4. What alternatives are there for treating eosinophilic esophagitis?

Dietary changes (elimination diets, elemental diets), pharmaceutical treatments (proton pump inhibitors, corticosteroids), endoscopic procedures (dilation, esophageal stents), allergy testing, and immunotherapy are possible treatment options for endoscopic oedema (EoE). Therapy selection is based on individual criteria, including patient preferences, treatment response, and the severity of the symptoms.

5. How can I regularly treat the symptoms of eosinophilic esophagitis?

Daily management of EoE symptoms may include eating an EoE-friendly diet, using prescription drugs as indicated, avoiding recognized triggers, maintaining excellent dental hygiene, and getting medical help quickly if symptoms worsen or flare up.

Reducing symptoms and enhancing quality of life can be achieved by establishing healthy lifestyle choices and collaborating closely with healthcare experts.

6. Are there resources for families and people suffering from eosinophilic esophagitis?

Yes, there are several support options available for people with Eosinophilic Esophagitis and their families, such as patient advocacy groups, online support groups, instructional websites, and local events. These tools help navigate the difficulties of living with EoE and interacting with members of the EoE community by offering knowledge, direction, and peer support.

www.ingramcontent.com/pod-product-compliance
Lightning Source LLC
Chambersburg PA
CBHW050813260726
48660CB00004B/1406